T0209934

A Vision of Healing

Healing

A Journey of Becoming Whole

WENDY FAIR WATERSON

WESTBOW
PRESS®
A DIVISION OF THOMAS NELSON
& ZONDERVAN

Unless otherwise indicated, all scripture taken from the New King James Version®.
Copyright © 1982 by Thomas Nelson. Used by permission. All rights reserved.

WestBow Press books may be ordered through booksellers or by contacting:

WestBow Press
A Division of Thomas Nelson & Zondervan
1663 Liberty Drive
Bloomington, IN 47403
www.westbowpress.com
1 (866) 928-1240

Because of the dynamic nature of the Internet, any web addresses or
links contained in this book may have changed since publication and
may no longer be valid. The views expressed in this work are solely those
of the author and do not necessarily reflect the views of the publisher,
and the publisher hereby disclaims any responsibility for them.

Any people depicted in stock imagery provided by Getty Images are
models, and such images are being used for illustrative purposes only.
Certain stock imagery © Getty Images.

ISBN: 978-1-9736-3905-3 (sc)
ISBN: 978-1-9736-3906-0 (e)

Print information available on the last page.

WestBow Press rev. date: 02/05/2019

Dedication

To my father, who first taught me about healing.
To my mother, who always prayed.

Acknowledgements

Many thanks to my husband, who cared for me in times of great need, always supported me in ministry, and also encouraged me to write. You are my hero! Love to my children, who have blessed me to be able to be that Mom who also did many other things. Thank you to all my family on both sides, who have assisted Chris and me in the tough moments, and especially those who have purposefully encouraged our dreams. Lots of love to my wonderful, powerful church family at Sanctuary Gate, now Shekhinah. You have sown into me and into this project in so many ways! Additional thanks and love to AP Teams. To all who have spoken the Word of the Lord over me throughout the years, I receive it, and thank you for being obedient to do so. Clearly He watches over it to perform it! I give thanks to Father God, precious Holy Spirit, and my Lord Jesus. You are my hope, life, and peace.

Contents

Introduction

I saw healing in a vision that I will never forget.

It was a vision that came in a dream as I was sleeping--but I felt awake. Suddenly I was on a sparkling beach under the sun with an ocean behind me, gazing up into brilliant blue sky. In a flash of movement of pure glowing white, a dove appeared high overhead.

It was coming straight to me. Somehow I believed it was also coming FOR me!

I found myself wondering that the wild bird would approach, and why, but I was ready to welcome it. In the dream I hoped it would land near me so I could view it from up close; but when the dove had almost reached me it was abruptly changed, instantly transformed into what I somehow knew in the dream to be a spirit. I also knew with an inner sense who this spirit was! It was the glorious Holy Spirit of God!!!

Holy Spirit came so close to me I could see nothing but Him hovering directly above my head. I was curiously impressed that He looked different than I had ever have imagined. It was as if He shimmered with manifestations of what I would call both feminine and masculine beauty, grace, strength and power!

A Vision of Healing

His being was full of a brightness that displayed glimpses of every color through it. I strained to see Him as He came very close. Suddenly I was conscious my vision through physical eyes was more blurred the nearer He came. I was highly disappointed by this! I absolutely wanted to see Him as clearly as possible, to drink in each detail about what He was like; however, in the dream my vision was imperfect like it was waking—a healing I had been praying for ever since I had developed vision problems several years earlier. In the dream I was aware of all of this, and remembered that I had decided to believe God to restore perfect vision to me. I had been waiting expectantly for it!

His hands reached out to gently encircle my face. Now He leaned very close to me so that all I could see were His eyes. As He gazed at me the intense light emanating from those eyes into mine was the brightest I had ever encountered! It surpassed the brilliance of the water, the glow of the sand, and somehow even the light of the sun in the sky behind Him. His light was more awesome than all of these! It was also clearer. It was purer. I was not afraid—He seemed so loving!

As the Spirit gazed closely at me I was again conscious that my vision was blurred, and that I could not perceive Him plainly because of it. As if reading my thoughts, and still looking deep into my eyes that needed healing, He spoke to me with a voice that I heard both within myself and outside myself. He clearly said, *"I'm going to fix that."*

Leaving the dream, and sleep as well, I felt more than physically awake. I felt awakened spiritually! I was excited by what I had seen and heard in this vision encounter!

"Lord," I said, "please show me what this means, and help

me to understand what You are revealing to me. I heard you say that You will fix my vision. Lord, I receive that." But somehow I knew He intended to do so much more!

I have been in an ongoing conversation with Father God through His Holy Spirit concerning healing, restoration and wholeness that has changed my life! There is remarkable transformation available to each of us through the Lord and His Spirit which includes healing of our bodies. It can come to us as we receive wisdom and understanding--a revelation of healing, and revelation of who the Lord is through gazing upon Him. May we each now be made whole, and the Lord receive all of the glory!

Chapter One: Devastation

I was 33 years old in 1995 when I was diagnosed with rheumatoid arthritis, and it exploded into my life suddenly, a dark and violent storm.

Newly pregnant with my third child Alyssa, I was occupied with baby preparations and not initially alarmed; however, before the pregnancy was over I would be in extreme pain and at times unable to walk. After a two month respite at the very end of the pregnancy and then one month just after she was born, I was not able to pick her up on my own. My husband would bring her to me so I could prop her on either arm and nurse her in bed or on the couch. When my baby was 3 ½ months old I gave up this way of feeding her instead of nursing her for 9 or 10 months as I had my first two children, Sarah and James. By the beginning of our third month together I was desperate for relief from pain. I accepted the strong medications the doctor recommended to me when I was first diagnosed but which I could not take at that time because I was expecting. Nursing was now out of the question.

I was devastated in my situation. Very ill and constantly suffering, I was now unable to nurse my child. I was facing the prospect of a lifetime of heavy medications. I learned my lifespan could be shortened by a decade or more because of the systemic nature of the disease. Finally, and worst of all in my mind, I was advised not to plan any more pregnancies.

I had always wanted to have four children! Now the rheumatologist said because of the medications I would need to take it would be best if I never became pregnant again. In response to the physician's counsel, my husband and I took measures so we would not have more children. My feeling of loss afterward was very great, and I deeply grieved our decision. My heart was broken.

One more blow to my soul was a statement my rheumatologist made that I would never forget: "You'll probably be in a wheelchair within five years."

My husband is my witness this actually happened. He was there with me in the doctor's examination room to hear it. To this day it seems out of place, and wrong, that a doctor would make this kind of declaration. Even 20 years ago strong medications typically kept arthritic patients from becoming crippled to the extent he was describing. Nevertheless, this was declared over me, at my first visit after initial diagnosis.

The words were powerful and paralytic by themselves. I saw myself in the wheelchair. Then I could also see my great-grandmother in memory from only a few visits with her before she passed. Her body was so crippled by arthritis she was frozen into a seated state. She wrote with difficulty, when a pen was placed into the space between her clenched fingers. I had been astonished at this as a child, and mildly horrified—but I played happily at her house with my cousins without further thought for Grandma's circumstances. Now I could distinctly imagine the pain she had suffered that must have accompanied the changed form of her body. I was feeling it myself.

I was trapped in a body that wasn't working, with a future of increasing pain and disability. I began to believe my life was over.

Fear is Torment

The medications I began to take after nursing my daughter for her first three and a half months made it possible for me to physically function a bit better, but they did not bring freedom from pain or remove the stiffness and inflammation. In fact, I remained very sick.

Darkness pressed in on me. I felt as though I was in a dream, as normal life began to fade. Some things that happened in those days—good things—I forgot. Things like my baby's first tooth, and when she walked. I was there, but I don't remember them. And I didn't record the milestones in her baby book as I had the other two children. I was too disturbed, too distracted. I was only trying to survive. The loss of these memories was a thing I cried over for many years.

Depression and fear began to take me over. Panic began to interrupt clear thought. Soon I felt unsafe going out or conducting daily business because of my state of mind.

Once during this time I ventured out to drive to a nearby city to see my youngest brother play a high school soccer game, but became lost on my way back. Somehow I couldn't gather my thoughts in order to find my way. I had always loved being on the road in a vehicle, and reading maps or driving alone was never a challenge. This time I barely made it home. I arrived a full hour after the time our eldest daughter, who was in kindergarten, was due to be dropped off by her school bus. In fear she was in danger or even missing after the long walk up our 600 foot driveway, I opened the door and rushed to the phone to call the school, hoping they had perhaps taken her back when I hadn't come to the door as I usually did. Then I heard her voice! She had let herself in with the spare key hidden outside our house. I didn't even know she knew where it was!

Fear is torment, and there are many costs to depression. During this time I begged my husband not to go to work because I was afraid to be home alone. My active life became restricted. When I did go out I heard voices cursing in my mind. I came to later believe there was a demonic element to what I experienced during that time. I believe satan saw my vulnerability, and sent demons to draw me further into that dark and desperate place.

Later I would be glad for my newborn and her need for me, though it was difficult to care for her, because I felt the commitment in my heart to that responsibility was a thing that kept me from taking my own life.

I expressed this to my parents when Mom and Dad came to visit to help and to bring encouragement. They looked shocked and sad when I said, "If I didn't have this baby I would go out in the field and kill myself." I regretted giving voice to it, and hoped they knew I didn't intend to wound their hearts, but the thought of peace and freedom from pain was inviting. I just wanted my agony to be over.

Chronic pain is something only those who have experienced it can understand, unless Holy Spirit somehow reveals it to someone who wants to know. For me in that season there seemed to be no other possibility of an end to my extreme distress. But in His goodness Father God had already intervened! I know now my new baby's presence in my life was truly a divine gift coming at just the right time. I know many were praying for me, especially Mom and Dad. And something more from the Lord was on the way!

Chapter Two: Can I Really Be Healed?

I n the midst of the severe illness it was my father who began to teach me about God's healing provision, a subject about which I knew nothing.

Sometime after I went away to college in the early 80's my father came into a personal revelation of healing. Now as he watched me in my desperate situation he determined to pass on to me what he had heard!

We lived 2 hours apart and Dad was not one to talk on the phone, but while I was ill he wrote to me often. Over the next few years he sent two or three notes or cards with healing Scriptures and insights every week. Day after day they were encouragement to believe God for that which I desperately needed! These words were precious, and they were lifelines I grasped at and tried my best to hold. I still have the cards to this day, although my father has gone on to be with the Lord in glory!

My father told me God was willing to heal me, and that this benefit was provided for me in Jesus. He wrote to me saying that fear had to go first, which I came to realize was a most profound statement! Then he introduced me to a healing Jesus, sending Scriptures like Matthew 8:16-17, *"When evening had come, they brought to Him many who were demon-possessed. And He cast out the spirits with a word, and healed all who were sick,[17]that it might be fulfilled which was spoken by Isaiah the prophet, saying:*

'He Himself took our infirmities, and bore our sicknesses.'"

Dad also taught me about faith. In one of his notes to me he wrote about how faith comes by hearing and grows over time. He said it was like learning to swim. First someone tells you it can be done, then you learn to float, and after that to dog paddle. At first you ease in, but later you dive in head first and swim under the water. He said in matters of faith few can jump right in. Many have been brought up with a mindset of fear—warned about how things might not work out rather than encouraged to believe for success and victory.

This described me exactly. I wanted to believe what Dad was saying to me. I could feel hope begin to come to me—and I hadn't felt that in a long time. But just as his note said, if faith was like jumping into the water, I wasn't ready.

I wasn't sure.

An Urgent Search

The concept of supernatural physical healing was uncomfortably unfamiliar to me, though I had given my life to Jesus, who my dad said was the Healer, in a very real experience at the age of 8. By 1995 when I first became ill I had been a believer in Him for 25 years. I considered Him my Savior. But no one had spoken to me about healing before I became ill, even once.

Wendy Fair Waterson

It seems odd now that in all the years of attending church, Vacation Bible School, and 6 years of Christian Junior High and High School this concept was never taught! When I went to college I was in church services from the very first Sunday I moved on campus until I graduated--nearly every Sunday throughout four years at college, and many times Wednesday nights as well for prayer. There was never a lesson given about healing. I do recall a few messages declaring miracles ceased with the age of the early church apostles.

I met my husband in that ministry I attended during college. We were happy there as a young married couple, and raised our little ones there among friends. Now, suddenly, in the face of the illness I had, I needed to know the Lord in a new way that they didn't speak about. I knew I needed this in order to survive! I desperately needed to know if I could be healed, and how to get it to happen. I began to pursue answers through every available avenue.

My search was hurried and stressful. I was starting from behind with almost no information, and having to now make up for lost time. I have always been grateful the illness I had wasn't immediately life threatening, or I could have died in the meantime! I purchased and read books about healing, and began to watch Christian television programming that spoke of it. I had never seen these kinds of shows before. I also started to visit a few ministries on Wednesday nights which seemed to believe in healing.

One church in town advertised healing prayer in the yellow pages, and I went to their afternoon healing clinic. No one else was there for prayer, but the minister was kind, and told me the depression and oppression I was experiencing was straight from satan, and the hopelessness in my mind was his attempt to paralyze me, convincing me things could never change. He called this the enemy's "smoke and mirrors." He prayed for me, but not really for healing. He prayed I would see and know the truth. He spoke as if addressing the enemy, and told him to leave me alone in the name of Jesus. After this visit some of the panic ceased.

In the midst of my search through media and ministries, I did not experience healing manifested immediately in my body; nevertheless, I realized God was changing things in my mind, just as the pastor at the healing clinic had prayed. My new experiences were good, and I found faith that healing was the will of God began to grow in my heart.

I Have Questions!

One Scripture often quoted by those I encountered who believed God would physically heal seemed to be a "go to" passage from the Bible on the matter. This key Scripture was 1 Peter 2:24, which is actually a quote of Isaiah 53:5.

> "... who Himself bore our sins in His own body on the tree, that we, having died to sins, might live for righteousness—by whose stripes you were healed."

> "But He was wounded for our transgressions, He was bruised for our iniquities; The chastisement for our peace was upon Him, And by His stripes we are healed."

I had never heard these verses used to reference physical healing before. These passages used for this purpose troubled my mind! Though nearly everyone who taught that physical healing could be expected from God seemed to rely on them, all I personally heard do so talked about it like it was so without explaining WHY. I wondered how anyone could conclude by these verses that the healing being discussed was actually physical healing.

Maybe the Scriptures in question only meant we were healed spiritually! After all, as believers in Jesus we do know we are forgiven, saved from sin, made new in Christ and restored to God. It's certainly an awesome spiritual healing God has worked for us in Jesus! Further, all might agree that spiritual healing would be the most important thing we could gain through salvation if we had to choose only one thing! We received forgiveness of sin and are bound for heaven! But was there actually "more" included? Was the healing meant to be physical also? If so, should I expect this?

This was something I very much needed to know! I apologized to the Lord that I was in this position of not being sure, praying, "Father, forgive me for asking for clarification about something maybe I should already know-- but if I'm going to believe you for this, I do have to know for sure!"

When you feel your life is at stake, you suddenly realize you need a true word! You need a solid anchor for your hope. You need the truth!

I began in depth study of the Scriptures. I knew I couldn't base my belief about God's willingness to heal or His provision for it for ME on anyone else's opinions or the results of their personal study unless I could clearly follow their progress through the word and understand their conclusion. I had to see the truth for myself, know that it came straight from the written word of God, and be assured that it was true by a confirmation through the Spirit. I could not base my faith for healing on an assumption. I needed a personal revelation.

He Will Give You Wisdom

Let me encourage you in a specific aspect of your relationship with God! He wants to answer your questions! This word is absolutely true that you can ask of Him and He will give you wisdom IN ABUNDANCE, WITHOUT SCOLDING YOU for asking! This is the truth of James 1:5, *"If any of you **lacks wisdom**, let him ask of God, who gives to all liberally and without reproach, and it will be given to him."*

I have relied on this characteristic of God many times! He knows I am a "question asker," but thankfully He is the Answer, and willing to share! True, I think I have heard Him say to me on occasion "You don't need to know that," but those times always involved a question about someone else's life. All were situations I quickly got the picture were none of my business! When asking about my own life, my direction, my need, He always seems so willing to share heavenly wisdom and knowledge to help me through. This is according to His character and His ways!

God is also not the author of confusion, so I have to believe He loves also to alleviate it, to clarify issues for us, and light our path with His word. That's Scripture! He is the Light that shines in our darkness!!! His word is a lamp to our feet, and it lights up our path (Psalm 119:105)! In our seeking He will always bring us back to His word to confirm what He is saying in our mind and spirit, and His word is His promise to us, because He *"is not a man that He should lie!"*

By the time I had received prayer for healing from others on several occasions, and had prayed for myself every day for months on end with no significant results, I began to pray specifically in a certain way that I believe was instrumental in my healing walk. I prayed, "Lord, please get me to the place where I CAN receive! Whatever You need to do in me, please do."

God honored that prayer. It was by teaching me through His Spirit and through His word that He answered me.

Taught by His Spirit: A Renewed Mind

Yes, the Lord took me deep into His word and taught me there by His Spirit!

It is important in whatever we are seeking from God to renew our thinking with His word and come to an understanding of His will. Discovering truth begins with a work in the heart and mind. If revelation is allowed to change our mind, transformation can occur; that is, the change we are seeking can come to us! This is a supernatural work of His Spirit. It won't happen any other way.

The book of Romans says, "... be transformed by the renewing of your mind," (vs. 12:2b). God's word through Scripture and through His Holy Spirit is what renews our mind! Then with the renewal, or a changed mind, we become candidates for transformation—including getting our bodies transformed or healed! His intention is that His word will change our thinking and enable us to receive all He has made available to us. His intention is our complete transformation!

All transformation, including healing, comes through agreement with God. It is easier to visualize how it can take place, or be blocked, if we define agreement as "alignment." Alignment simply means "an adjustment to a line."

Alignment is important. Being in alignment "lines you up" to receive! If the provision you are seeking from heaven is like a waterfall, alignment means standing under it. If you don't stand under it, you won't get very wet! If you do stand under it, or align your mind with the word of God about something, you can then fully receive it! Line up with God's word, and then let the word of God deluge your spirit, soul and body!

Be Honest, Ask for Grace!

Do you know what Scripture says concerning healing, whether emotional, spiritual, or physical? Honesty is important! If we don't know what is in the word, or if a specific thing in it is unknown to us, it may take some time to have a manifestation of transformation. It takes time to have our mind renewed! Admitting we don't know something is a first critical step towards receiving life transforming new revelation.

If you are in the same place of uncertainty that I was, ask for grace from the Lord and press in. Open your heart and ask God to show you the truth about what He has given you in Jesus. Holy Spirit will take the truth in Scripture and quicken it, or bring it to life, inside of you. He will confirm these truths with His present word spoken into your spirit and soul, until your mind, will and emotions are each renewed and changed!!! Once you have revelation of God's will on an issue or problem, you will be able to believe and trust Him to bring the answer to you, knowing it is surely in His heart to do it!

Wendy Fair Waterson

When He "Hears," We Have It!

I AM CONVINCED the Lord wants us to be healed even more than we want to be. It's a matter of His love for us and his integrity. His willingness to help me discover the truth in my journey towards healing itself was evidence of His desire. Looking back I realize how very much the Lord was for me in my seeking! The supernatural began to unfold in my life in significant ways as Holy Spirit worked to bring revelation I needed and was requesting from Him.

I had read the Bible all my life and not received a personal revelation of healing, but then I had not been seeking! After I asked to know, the Scriptures began to open up to me in a new way.

Holy Spirit quickened 1 John 5:14-15 to me early in my learning process. This word says, *"Now this is the confidence that we have in Him, that if we ask anything according to His will, He hears us. And if we know that He hears us, whatever we ask, we know that we have the petitions that we have asked of Him."*

I began to realize that if I was going to receive any one thing from God, including healing, it was truly going to have to be a case where I *knew* it was God's will. The remarkable thing was that this Scripture said how I could know He would say yes to my request! He would say yes to anything that was His will! If it was His will He would then "hear"...and if He "heard" He would grant the request. In fact, and even more remarkably, if what I had asked was His will I would know I not only *could* have, but *did* have the thing I had asked for given to me! Anything that is God's will has essentially already been given. *"...if we know that He hears us, whatever we ask, we know that we **have** the petitions* *that we have asked of Him."* The only thing that remains is for us to receive it!

This kind of truth from Scripture is the beginning of alignment concerning healing principles. The simple and necessary understanding of His will in the matter is foundational for a healing revelation, or any other. After all, if a thing isn't God's will, why bother asking? Grasping hold of the truth of 1 John 5:14 and 15 and adding to it other Scriptures that indicate healing IS His will can bring us out of doubt and into a positive faith that receives.

So, was healing God's will for me?

Chapter Three: He said, "Yes!"

"By His stripes we are healed."

In my quest for understanding I asked the Lord for explanation of this curious word from Scripture. I wanted to believe this meant what some people said—that the beating and death Jesus endured on the cross bought freedom from sickness, disease, and the distressing pain I experienced every day and every night. My salvation through Jesus was vividly real to me. Certainly no one could ever have talked me out of it. I had known beyond doubt, since I was a girl of eight, I was saved from sin and hell--but I knew nothing of any kind of physical healing provision. I had no hope for healing in my body when I became ill, or in the early days of my study of healing through the Bible.

One Word Study Will Help You

One of the most significant seasons of revelation came when the Spirit taught me concerning the very Scripture I struggled to understand. He revealed transforming truth from 1 Peter 2:24 and Isaiah 53:5! To the present time the revelation through these

A Vision of Healing

verses is one of the most compelling indications to me of how surely we can each know we have been provided physical healing through Jesus' sacrifice for us!

A single word study from the Isaiah passage reveals what is inherent in the original word translated "healed." This is the word *raphah* (raw-faw') defined in Strong's Exhaustive Concordance (#7495) this way: to mend by stitching, to cure, cause to heal, physician, repair, (thoroughly), make whole. [1]

It is used in more than 60 Scripture verses which describe a wide variety of things as "healed." These include people, the nation of Israel, injury, sickness, and objects that have been broken or damaged. That such a variety of things are called "healed" is indicative of the true meaning of the word and its root.

Hebrew can be understood more clearly by looking at the root word for the word in question. *Rapha* comes from the root *rwp*, or *rp²*, which rightly means "to restore to normal."[3] The tense of this verb healed, is perfect, revealing that whatever healing is indicated has, in fact, already been done. It means something has been put back in its original form. It has been fixed or repaired. It has been made whole again. As we have been assured "it is finished!"[4] (John 19:30).

The meaning of the word *raphah* is a key to understanding the revelation through Isaiah 53:5, and consequently I Peter 2:24,

---

1. Strong's Exhaustive Concordance #7495.

2. Ibid.

3. W.E. Vine, M.F. Unger, and W. White Jr., An Expository Dictionary of Biblical Words, (Nashville: Thomas Nelson Publishers,1984), s.v., "healing."

4. Brown, Francis, S. R. Driver, and Charles A. Briggs, A Hebrew and English Lexicon of the Old Testament, (Oxford: Clarendon Press, 1906. Reprint, 1951).

and to knowing the place physical healing has in God's plan for His redeemed people!

Here is how it works: Through Jesus suffering and then His death on the cross we have been spiritually reconciled to God or restored (2 Corinthians 5:18). God the Father has brought us to Himself in Christ and has forgiven our sin which had previously separated us from Him. This process has now returned us to our original state mankind enjoyed before sin entered into the earth. We are now restored to God!

Ultimately, I came to view I Peter 2:24 and Isaiah 53:5 in this way: "By His stripes we have been forgiven and restored!" Further, in that place of restoration we have everything! Healing in Jesus isn't "spiritual, but not physical." It is physical *because* it is spiritual! Being completely restored to the Father, you could not receive one without the other. You absolutely get both!

As I saw this reality and internalized it, great relief flooded my mind, and the darkness in my soul significantly lifted. I felt I could now accept what the people who spoke of healing wanted to tell me and others—by His stripes we are healed---not only spiritually, but physically!

I began to pray to be healed this way. I began to believe it could happen. I began to say aloud, "I've been forgiven and restored!"

Chapter Four: But When?

A fter the Lord answered my question of whether He was willing to heal me, I had another question!

(You knew that I would!)

I had asked and been answered concerning, "Can I be healed?" Now I needed to know when!

I prayed, "Lord, when is healing? When can we actually be healed?" I very much needed to know the answer, as I struggled day to day to get up in the morning and take care of my family. I was encouraged by what I was learning about God and His healing power, and I had come to believe He was willing to release healing to me, but it didn't seem to be here yet. I found this to be discouraging, and also odd, as there seemed no good reason for it since I needed healing NOW.

I thought, "If I was tied up on a railroad track and a train was coming, when do I need to be rescued? NOW!" If you have ever been extremely sick, you might identify with my feelings!

By now two years had passed since the diagnosis I was given. I and my family had relocated into a Spirit-baptized church setting, and were surrounded by people who believed in healing.

A Vision of Healing

This can be helpful in and of itself, as you will benefit from sitting under healing teaching, hearing testimonies, and worshiping with music that declares God's healing power. Still, I was disappointed to discover MANY of the people still referred to healing as something that would eventually happen in their future. "I know the Lord will heal me someday," they would say. "In His timing."

I prayed long and hard about this. It seemed so wrong!! Never in Scripture in the accounts where Jesus healed did He ever ask someone to wait! Surely there should have been one example of that if it were an option that He for some reason cared to use!

Jesus only did what He saw the Father doing. Evidently He never saw Him waiting to release healing!! Once He seems to have stopped in process with a healing half finished, in the healing of the blind man in Mark 8:22-25. In the midst of ministering to the man Jesus asked him, *"Do you see anything,"* and he reported *"I see men like trees, walking."* It was as if the healing had partially come and the man had regained some sight, but not all. Then Jesus touched him a second time and the man could see clearly. Notice in the account Jesus did not wait to minister the healing, only to finish, and the finishing caused no apparent distress, as it was then immediately completed.

I am convinced that performing this healing in two parts was not necessary; however, I believe it was done intentionally and purposefully in this way, and put in Scripture as such, to illustrate a specific scenario where healing might be delayed for some external reason (outside of God's clear will to heal). Note that Jesus took the man and led him out of the town to minister to him. I believe He did this in order to have freedom to perform the miracle just this way, without onlookers having reason to comment afterwards, "He could not do it at first!"

Wendy Fair Waterson

This account where the man's sight is restored in two parts is an encouragement that even if healing for some reason comes as a process, it is the will of the Lord to heal! That can be our first assumption. Our second assumption, unless the Lord says for a specific and legitimate reason it will be otherwise, should be that healing will take place immediately. Delay of full healing could occur if there isn't a full faith to receive, or if some other issue were to arise. If a healing today is delayed, we can pray to know the reason, and address it.

Where my own healing was concerned I believed early on that if God wanted me to wait He should, and would, inform me of the fact. That I should wait was not an assumption I was willing to make without a clear word saying so--and a word from Him, not from anyone else!

I decided to use my faith for an answer to the question of when I could be healed.

I asked this of the Lord for my own sake, but also shared my heart with Him in preparation for a future of sharing His word with others. "Lord," I said, "Please tell me clearly and tell me right! Because whatever you say to me is what I am going to say to every person I ever come across in this life who needs to be healed."

I heard from Him.

"I Will Tell You Tomorrow".

I was sitting on my bed on a Saturday night asking my question when I heard the Spirit say it clearly. *"I will tell you tomorrow."*

Have you ever heard the beautiful voice of Holy Spirit? It was the first time that I had heard Him in this way, like a voice nearly audible, speaking both within me and just beside me at the same time. I can't describe to you fully how you will know when it is He who speaks, but you will know that you know!

I was thrilled by the experience—and with the answer! I was going to know tomorrow!

But why not today?

God does not toy with us. He is not playing games with our emotions! And rather than demanding we jump through certain hoops to be healed I believe He is trying to find the best way for each of us to receive. I think He is looking for the easiest way to get our healing to us!

If He says to you, "Go receive prayer at the Benny Hinn meeting," it's not for fun on His part, but because He needs to get you to a place where you can be healed. Do whatever He says to do! He wants you to be well! He knows how you can best receive! And He knows places where the anointing of the Spirit is flowing to heal! He is not making you do things for His own entertainment.

I believe one reason He had me wait until the next day to hear an answer was because the way He would do it was about to be remarkable enough for me to be sure. I would need to recall the word He would give and be convinced it was true when it was later tested by contrary circumstances. I was going to need to know it was from Him, and rely on it through difficult days. His word and these prophetic experiences would become sign posts towards which I would move, keeping them in sight when I was weary. I also believe this communication from Him was geared especially for me to be able to receive. Remember that I had been praying, "Lord, whatever you need to do in me to cause me to be able to receive, please do it."

"I will tell you tomorrow." I fell asleep with this precious word close in my heart.

"Tomorrow" was Sunday, and I was going to our local church gathering.

Chapter Five:
Healing is Now!!!

I t was a small but vibrant Assembly of God church to which we had relocated by an invitation "out of the blue" from someone my husband and I hadn't heard from in a number of years. They invited us to a picnic at a Pentecostal church they themselves didn't even attend—"The Lord said to call and invite you to come. We don't even go there, we're just going for the day." By now we had still been attending only a few weeks. I was about to find out the reason for the unusual manner in which we had come to be here. It was a heavenly set up!

The meeting began and I was all ears. The Lord's word to me from the night before was all I had on my mind.

On this Sunday the musicians and vocalists began praising and worshiping the Lord as they usually did at the start of a meeting. I loved the freedom of their worship and the joyful praise they expressed week to week. I found I wanted to be in a place where hands were raised in honor of the Lord when I found out my God was willing to heal!

A Vision of Healing

Sitting in my seat, then standing to worship, I reminded the Lord what I had prayed—how that I wanted and *needed* to know, "When is healing?" I also reminded Him I planned to use His answer whenever the question arose in the future with ANYONE else who was ill and wanted to know. I believed we had a deal, and an understanding.

The instant the worship team began to sing I knew the answer was truly here!

"This is the Day of the Favor of the Lord" the words said. It was a song by Lindell Cooley out of the Brownsville revival. I had come late into the revival, and the song was new to me, but I was clearly hearing it now! I knew undoubtedly this was the answer to my question, and the answer He intended me to hear when He said on Saturday, *"I will tell you tomorrow."* Now, today, He was saying, *"**This** is the day."*

I was in awe of God!!! From that moment of the meeting everything that took place that day, including the pastor's sermon, was about the one message: "Today."

In hindsight it is no surprise that this was the answer and the word the Lord gave to me! Even a cursory, if open-minded, reading of Scripture reveals the truth about *today* with God!

Here is what the written word of God says in confirmation of my experience. Some of these verses were in the message I heard so many years ago. By now they are key passages I might use for anyone asking the same question I did, but in 1997 this application of them was entirely new. If you have not heard them this way, you may say as I did, "Why didn't I see it before?"

Wendy Fair Waterson

Today is the Day of Salvation!

> *For He says: "In an acceptable time I have heard
> you, and in **the day of salvation** I have helped
> you." Behold, now **is the** accepted time; behold,
> now **is the day of salvation.*** 2 Corinthians 6:2*

The apostle Paul quotes from Isaiah 49:8-9, a prophetic picture of the time in which the Lord Jesus would come and manifest His deliverance for His people Israel and show His favor upon them among the nations in a tangible manner. For them it was a day yet to come...but then Paul says, "But look, the time is actually here!!!" *"Behold, now **is the** accepted time; behold, now **is the day of salvation.**" (2 Corinthians 6:2b)* There is strong emphasis given that those receiving this word should pay diligent attention and TAKE NOTICE! "Behold" is given twice—"Look, and look again!!!"

Jesus came and died and was raised, and in these ways, along with the ministry He performed during His time on earth, He finished the work He was given to do (John 17:4). Now Paul confirms even to the believers of his day that the day of salvation is *fully* come. Yes, even at that time there was to be no more waiting! So it is for us today—for all who believe.

We can believe salvation is for today and stake our lives and our healings upon it! In fact, the Spirit of the Lord through Paul pleads with us in 2 Corinthians 6:1-2 not to miss out on this reality!

> *We then, as workers together with Him also **plead
> with you not to receive the grace of God in vain.**
> ²For He says: "In an acceptable time I have heard*

A Vision of Healing

*you, and in the day of salvation I have helped you." Behold, now **is the** accepted time; behold, now is the day of salvation.*

The Spirit urges us to receive <u>today,</u> and not let the gift of salvation, and all that it includes, escape us!

Today is the Day of God's Favor!

So He came to Nazareth, where He had been brought up. And as His custom was, He went into the synagogue on the Sabbath day, and stood up to read. ¹⁷And He was handed the book of the prophet Isaiah. And when He had opened the book, He found the place where it was written:
¹⁸"The Spirit of the LORD is upon Me,
Because He has anointed Me
To preach the gospel to the poor;
He has sent Me to heal the brokenhearted,[i]
To proclaim liberty to the captives
And recovery of sight to the blind,
To set at liberty those who are oppressed;
¹⁹To proclaim the acceptable year of the LORD."[k]
²⁰Then He closed the book, and gave it back to the attendant and sat down. And the eyes of all who were in the synagogue were fixed on Him. ²¹And He began to say to them, "Today this Scripture is fulfilled in your hearing." Luke 4:16-21

Jesus picked up the scroll and read from Isaiah 61:1-2a, and said that the Isaiah Scripture was fulfilled! He said *"I came to preach under the anointing of the Spirit of the Lord, and to set everyone free from any kind of affliction or bondage. I came to proclaim the time when God's favor comes upon all men—the year of the favor of the Lord!"*

He said, *"I came to do it, and I <u>am</u> doing it. Today this Scripture is fulfilled in your hearing."* In other words, *"The time is here!"*

Scriptures like these were, and are, powerful confirmations to me of a revelation of Today healing! Jesus' own testimony confirming His purpose in the earth settles the issue for all who can receive the truth of it. What could keep us in captivity in a day when He has made us free? **It's time for our prison stay to be over.** Whatever bondages have been holding us can be expected to break, through the anointing Jesus has released into our lives by His presence and work.

As I began to perceive what He had done for me, I began to pray receiving prayers.

Lord, I thank you that in Jesus I have complete freedom from every affliction or binding thing. I was captive, but I have been released. I was broken, but am now healed; I was blind, but I see! In Jesus all this that was written is fulfilled, and I receive it! AMEN.

Praise Jesus!

Today is the Day of His Rest!

A revelation of God's rest can also move you into healing.

The writer of Hebrews tells an intriguing, but troubling story about the nation of Israel who had been promised a land flowing with milk and honey as a place to live. By a miraculous deliverance they escaped Egypt, then traveled through the wilderness toward the good place promised to them in the word spoken beforehand.

A Vision of Healing

Unfortunately, Scripture reports (as we referenced before) they then failed to mix the word they had received with faith. *Hebrews 4:2b "...but the word which they heard did not profit them, not being **mixed with faith** in those who heard it."* Because of this, they did not enter the land of the promise. In fact, the generation actually given the promise died in the wilderness--except, of course, the two spies who brought back the good report—Joshua and Caleb!

Next, Scripture says this vacuum of belief created an interesting situation; namely, "*... a promise remains of entering His rest...*" *Hebrews 4:1a*

I love this quality of our God! He is not going to let a good thing go to waste! He intends for His blessings to be blessing someone! Here God has a rest prepared, and He highly desires someone to access it! He is interested in fulfilling His own promise, and is looking for people who will reach for it and obtain it. I want one of them to be me!

> *Since therefore it remains that some must enter it, and those to whom it was first preached did not enter because of disobedience, ⁷again He designates a certain day, saying in David, "Today," after such a long time, as it has been said:*
> *"Today, if you will hear His voice,*
> *Do not harden your hearts."*
> *⁸For if Joshua had given them rest, then He would not afterward have spoken of another day. ⁹There remains therefore a rest for the people of God.*
> *Hebrews 4:6-8*

Of course the promised land of Canaan was a picture of a

Wendy Fair Waterson

spiritual reality that would ultimately be found in Jesus Christ Himself—the true and complete rest found in the promise of salvation in Him! Perfect rest is in Jesus!

The writer of Hebrews makes it clear that the call of God has always been to draw His people into rest and peace, and that anyone in their own time could begin walk into that reality, though it would certainly only come to its fullness in Jesus. But now He has come and finished His work! The promise of rest still exists, and now can surely be fully entered! If we would hear and enter, we could come into it!

When is the promise valid and accessible? *"Today."* The Today of God is in Jesus. The Today of God IS Jesus! Have you received Him? If so, this rest is for you, and includes all He has provided through His death on the cross.

Good To Go!

The Spirit in this season is trying to move us into a place of full understanding of all that we have been given through Jesus! He is speaking this in His Church, as well as to those who don't yet know Him personally. The message is that everything that is God's will for us is already in Him, coming to us in the package that is our salvation. Because of this provision Father God says to us that when we ask something that is in His will we may rightly consider not only that He will give it, but that it is already ours through His provision in Christ!

One day while home alone praying on my couch I had an interesting conversation with the Lord that put the seal on my knowledge of His will being for my healing, as well as the appropriate timing of it in God's eyes. It was as if the door to doubt had been open yet a little. That day it slammed shut.

33

A Vision of Healing

I remember that my young son was playing in the next room as I sat on the sofa praying. Like so many days at that time I was torn by sharp pain throughout my body. Wellness for people with arthritis is measured by quality of sleep, how long morning stiffness lasts, and the number of swollen and tender joints one has (among other technical measures). In my case, nearly all my joints were involved. I ached all over. During the first year of onset I was also diagnosed with fibromyalgia which added to my suffering. I attended a seminar at a hospital on people who had both. I remember a slide they displayed that said 80% of people with both rheumatoid arthritis and fibromyalgia eventually lived as invalids. Oh, yes, in those days my outlook in the natural, without God, was grim.

"Father," I cried, "I hurt so badly! I don't understand why I still have not been healed, but I really need You to answer my questions. I know this can't be Your fault, but must be because of something to do with me. I need help!"

Then I thought of all the people who said they'd seen the Lord and spoken with Him. I was suddenly angry with God that I had not had this happen for me! I had not had a time when He appeared in MY room and spoke to me, telling me what His will was and then taking away my sickness the way He did in the accounts in the New Testament or in amazing stories of miracles in the present day.

I called out loud to God, "I can't do this anymore! And You need to **come down here** and talk to me. You need to come and tell me what your will is for My healing! You need to answer my questions!!"

Like a surge of a tide or a sudden wind, the Spirit welled up in and around me. I was impressed deep within that the Lord said very firmly four clear words.

He said, "*I already did that.*"

It took me up short! I was grateful that He spoke, but also astounded that is what He said!

I am convinced the Lord is willing to tell us things more than once, or appear before us in a spiritual encounter; but on that day and in that way He was releasing to me another new revelation. It was emphasized most pointedly by His NOT appearing in front of me in my room! This is what I believe He said:

> *"I already sent Jesus down there! And through His ministry, death and resurrection for you He already spoke My will in this matter. He showed you not only My intentions, but what I have in fact already DONE."*

I have learned not to be offended with the Lord's adjustments to my thinking. They are always profitable! Further, I have found His chosen method and manner of speaking, whenever it occurs, are supremely wise, and always the very best! He speaks intentionally, and not one word or accompanying action of His is wasted. Even His silence is there can be message that can be interpreted to us by His Spirit!

Congruent to when He pointedly refused to "come down here" are several specific moments He declined to discuss my healing—perhaps as many times as those moments when He answered a prayer for insight almost immediately. I have had times I was thinking of my healing and nothing else during prayer, petitioning the Lord for it, when to my surprise He began to talk to me about something completely different! I came to believe this was really His way of saying. *"We don't need to talk about it! Remember? You're good to go!"*

Today is the day of healing! *A promise remains of entering His rest...and some must enter it.* WHAT ABOUT YOU? What about now?

Chapter Six: More Proofs of Healing

My personal study of healing, from its beginning to the point I could pray, ask and believe to receive it, took nine months. Perhaps it was in itself like a pregnancy and birth, but one of a different, spiritual kind! The word had to enter my heart as a seed and grow until it could produce its fruit—a harvest of healing. Eventually I decided to take God at His word. I chose to believe that what He said, including *"By His stripes we are healed"* was true! My health began to change.

I hope what you have read so far has SAVED you at least 9 months of study! Ask the Lord in prayer to confirm to you what is from Him and is the truth. He will answer you!

Following are three additional and specific ways Father God spoke to me and led me, helping me embrace His healing truth. They are very simple, but each played its part to give me hope and understanding of God's ways and His heart towards each of us!

A Vision of Healing

ONE: The Lord reminded me how our bodies are created with the capacity to heal.

The body will heal itself if given a chance.

Look at the scrape or cut on your finger. Within seconds, blood cells close off the wound, then harden to cover it so that tender new skin cells can form and multiply. Within just a few short days the wound is closed. You think nothing of it, because you have seen this amazing process occur so often. And yet, isn't it the stuff of creative miracles? New skin is formed over a hole in flesh!

The body naturally fights against germs and viruses. Given sufficient nutrition and proper rest, remarkable recoveries are made every day without calling the healing team!

Wouldn't it be strange if Father God, our Creator, didn't want us healed but had made each of our bodies to be remarkably self-healing? If the Lord had no interest in alleviating pain and suffering, why would He arrange our nervous system so that the sensation of rubbing our body where pain exists actually works? The soft touch reaches our brain and is interpreted as feeling good before the sensation of pain can be transferred and interpreted. The transmission of the sensation of pain is blocked by the surge of soothing touch from other, bigger nerve pathways--all by God's own design! He is interested in relieving suffering.

I find it interesting that no one questions God's will for us to be healed from daily scrapes and bruises and minor sicknesses, but His will comes into question concerning more extensive problems. In the first set of circumstances we never doubt we're going to fully recover, but in the next suddenly our potential for healing is a great mystery.

Wendy Fair Waterson

Once during the time I was just beginning to learn about the healing God had provided for me, I experienced His concern over my pain in a remarkable manner. Scripture reveals that angels are sent to minister to us, those who have inherited salvation (Hebrews 1:14), and I believe one was sent to me!

At times with arthritis the pain becomes so severe sleep will not come. I had a habit of moving to the couch to sit up if this happened, and on a certain night I had gone downstairs into our family room, the back room of the house, to try to rest. I struggled for hours to find a comfortable position, but when I began to drift off in sleep the pain always returned. Desperate, I prayed to the Lord for relief. Half asleep, I would inevitably feel the pain coming again.

The room had been dark, and the hall that led to it as well. I prayed, a little bit out of my new level of revelation, but mostly in desperation in the moment: "Lord, please help me. I just want to sleep."

With my eyes closed, I saw the door opened and light coming down the hallway. Then I felt my body be lifted up and repositioned on the couch, just so. Afterwards I slept until morning!

I will always testify that our Father cares for us. He hears us when we call. I know from experience that the Lord is continually with us in difficulty, and is working in every troubled situation to bring us out. I know that He is willing to remove our pain. He is willing to use any means within His holy and righteous respository to bring about our deliverance.

He wants us to be well!

A Vision of Healing

TWO: The Lord highlighted for me the one account in the Bible where a person asked Jesus if He was willing to heal him—and Jesus said, "I am willing."

There is a principle in study of Scripture called the Law of First Mention. By it we study any biblical doctrine by going to the reference where that thing is first mentioned, and studying it there in it foundational form. Where a thing or concept is first mentioned, it carries special, weighty significance. In the case of a man with leprosy in Luke 5 and Mark 1 it is a first and singular account of someone asking what so many want to know, "Is God willing to heal me?".

> *And it happened when He was in a certain city, that behold, a man who was full of leprosy saw Jesus; and he fell on his face and implored Him, saying, "Lord, if You are willing, You can make me clean." Then He put out His hand and touched him, saying, "I am willing; be cleansed." Immediately the leprosy left him.*
> *Luke 5:12-13*

The man wanted to know if Jesus would heal HIM, not if He was just generally willing to heal people. This is a question nearly everyone who is sick and comes to God wants to know! Today, just as in the New Testament account, the answer from the God who does not change is surely, *"Yes, I am willing!"*

The Scriptural account goes on to say that MULTITUDES came to Jesus for healing as a result of this event. The Savior asked the man not to spread the word, but he did!

However, the report went around concerning Him all the more; and great multitudes came together to hear, and to be healed by Him of their infirmities. Luke 5:15

I am thinking it was because they all heard not only that He was able to heal, but that He was also willing! They came, not just to hear, but to be healed!

THREE: The Lord showed me in Scripture the pattern of Jesus in ministering physical healing was to heal all who asked.

There are four accounts where Jesus literally healed all the sick who were present (Matthew 8:16-17, Matthew 12:15, Luke 4:38-40, Luke 6:19), and other references that do not use the word "all," but describe a scenario where many were brought to be healed and "He healed their sick." Although we do not find the Bible explicitly states that He always healed all who were there, there are reasons for Him not doing so that are consistent with His greater desire to do so-- if He is not obstructed. One of them is that sometimes the people present did not receive Him, so could not in faith receive what He brought. Scripture records that in Jesus' home town of Nazareth:

When He had come to His own country, He taught them in their synagogue, so that they were astonished and said, "Where did this Man get this wisdom and these mighty works? 55 Is this not the carpenter's son? Is not His mother called Mary? And His brothers James, Joses, Simon, and Judas?56 And His sisters, are they not all with us?

A Vision of Healing

Where then did this Man get all these things?"[57]So they were offended at Him. But Jesus said to them, "A prophet is not without honor except in his own country and in his own house."[58]Now He did not do many mighty works there because of their unbelief. Matthew 13:54-58

One thing is abundantly clear! In the biblical accounts He *always* responded with healing *whenever* anyone asked for it! The weight of that evidence is compelling! Scripture records that Jesus was manifested for a purpose, and that was to destroy the works of the devil (1 John 3:8); then He immediately went out into the streets, and across the countryside illustrating what that looked like. This is wonderful, because it looked like all kinds of healing and deliverance!

A case for healing can be made from Jesus' response to demon possession as well. He treated sickness and demons both the same, as things to be removed when encountered. We see no difference in His attitude towards the two issues. He went where the Father sent Him, doing what the Father said to do, and setting people free from every kind of afflicting thing.

If you are requesting healing from the Lord, the clear pattern of Scripture reveals that He will say, *"Yes!"* The same Jesus who healed over 2,000 years ago lives today to heal and set us free!

The overwhelming evidence in the written word of God for healing is supported by the patterns of ministry of Jesus, as well as evidence in the natural world. Our Creator God, our Father in heaven, is very willing for each of us to be healed and whole!

Wendy Fair Waterson

There is Healing in the Word, and All the Word Heals!

In a very real sense, all Scripture points to Jesus or directly speaks about Him. Jesus is the Word and the word is also the Scripture. If Jesus is healing (and He is), then all Scripture is eventually connected to healing!

Healing is a thread throughout the tapestry of God's word—or perhaps the entire tapestry could be titled "All that is God"--including healing. If I drape the tapestry over me, the healing thread touches me! This concept of healing being inherent in the entire word of God is a truth that will encourage your heart and inspire you as you study the whole counsel of the written word—the entire Holy Bible.

Many books are available that extensively list healing Scriptures. I will focus on those that have been most helpful to me. Some of them can be considered foundation, or very basic and obvious references to healing, and others are those from which healing can be rightly extrapolated or inferred. They are all a blessing!

Psalm 103:1-5

This passage takes us back to the basics of what God has done for us in Jesus, declaring plainly that our God does, indeed, forgive our iniquities and heal our diseases—all of them.

> *Bless the LORD, O my soul;*
> *And all that is within me, bless His holy name!*
> *²Bless the LORD, O my soul,*
> *And forget not all His benefits:*
> *³Who forgives all your iniquities,*
> *Who heals all your diseases,*

A Vision of Healing

⁴Who redeems your life from destruction,
Who crowns you with lovingkindness and tender
mercies,
⁵Who satisfies your mouth with good things,
So that your youth is renewed like the eagle's.

The point made in an earlier chapter that our spiritual healing effectively produces the physical is beautifully supported here! There is the consistent progression from deliverance from sin to freedom from disease.

I love that David is speaking to himself in this Psalm, doing as Scripture describes he would sometimes do, strengthening himself in the Lord his God! He reminds himself of God's provision, because, like us, he tends to forget. David sets before himself for consideration ALL the benefits the Father has bestowed upon him. He meditates on them, and rehearses them aloud.

Jehovah God has forgiven David's iniquities and healed his diseases—every one. He has redeemed David's life from destruction. Finally, it is no insignificant state of affairs that results from this redemption! David ends up *crowned* with God's love, kindness and mercy, and miraculously having his youth renewed by the power of the Lord! I believe David valued this crown made up of God's lovingkindness and tender mercies more than the one marking him as king of a nation. And, by the way, who would want the one without the other?

As always with the Lord, we get it all—wholeness in body soul and spirit, AND the fulfillment of our call and destiny in the earth! The crowning in this passage is a prophetic image of everything we have been given in our redemption through Christ. This access to God's goodness is what everyone receives whose sin is forgiven!

Wendy Fair Waterson

Job 33:23-26

If I were to choose a favorite healing passage, this wonderful one might be my top choice. Because the book of Job was disturbing to me as usually preached, I spent a season allowing Holy Spirit to speak to me about its message.

Job contains premium healing revelation. It is striking when finally understood and laid against the norm.

You've probably heard of Job's three friends. They have an awful reputation for being accusers, and blaming Job for his troubles. However, there was a fourth friend! For some reason Elihu is not nearly so famous--but he should be! Below are the words of Job's fourth friend as he declares the provision of God available to Job if he will access it:

> *If there is a messenger for him,*
> *A mediator, one among a thousand,*
> *To show man His uprightness,*
> *24Then He is gracious to him, and says,*
> *'Deliver him from going down to the Pit;*
> *I have found a ransom';*
> *25His flesh shall be young like a child's,*
> *He shall return to the days of his youth.*
> *26He shall pray to God, and He will delight in him,*
> *He shall see His face with joy,*
> *For He restores to man His righteousness.*

Here is a paraphrase. (Note that I wrote this paraphrase, and without influence from any other paraphrase. I recommend doing this from time-to-time in order to build understanding of a passage through expressing the ideas personally!):

45

A Vision of Healing

Job 33:23-26, paraphrased: "If a man is dying, may he be fortunate enough to find someone who will be his mediator, to take a message from him to God, and bring one back from God to the man. If the mediator can convince the dying man that it is God's righteousness and not his own that can save him, then God will graciously give the word, *'Deliver him! Do not allow him to be punished through death! A ransom has been given for him through the one who came as his mediator!'* Then watch what happens to the dying man! He will become healthy again in his body, and his youth will even be restored! The man will pray, and the Lord will show him how delighted He is with him. The joy of the Lord will shine from the Lord's face upon that man! It's all because He has placed His own righteousness upon the man who was dying—a righteousness that restores him in every way!"

When the Job passage is examined in light of what our Lord Jesus has done, it is evident that Jesus is the mediator who has brought about the release of our healing!

The point seems to have escaped us that Job, though noted as being without sin in the beginning of the book, eventually erred by presenting his own righteousness to God as the reason he should not be allowed to suffer. Three friends accused him of sinning, but offered the wrong solution—just stop sinning. But it was never about Job's sin or lack of sin. Into the story comes the fourth friend—I believe a representation of Jesus Christ—to release the truth.

> *Surely you have spoken in my hearing,*
> *And I have heard the sound of your words, saying,*
> *'I am pure, without transgression;*
> *I am innocent, and there is no iniquity in me.*

[10]Yet He finds occasions against me,
He counts me as His enemy;
[11]He puts my feet in the stocks,
He watches all my paths.'
[12]"Look, in this you are not righteous.
I will answer you,
For God is greater than man. Job 33:8-12

The last friend points out the truth of where Job went wrong. By holding up his own righteous living as meriting salvation, he became unrighteous (verse 12). Like Job we must look to God only to be qualified for His provision and salvation, "for God is greater than man."

This passage from Job has been life-giving to me, and highly instrumental to my understanding that I have been restored to God and healed!

Here are more passages I have loved concerning healing:

- *Psalm 91* (all of it!)

- *Colossians 1:13 "He has **delivered us** from the power of darkness and **conveyed us** into the kingdom of the Son of His love..."*

- *Matthew 9:20-22 "And suddenly, a woman who had a flow of blood for twelve years came from behind and touched the hem of His garment.[21] For she said to herself, "If only I may touch His garment, I shall be made well."[22]But Jesus turned around, and when He saw her He said, 'Be of good cheer, daughter; your faith has made you well.'And the woman was made well from that hour."* (with *Matthew 14:35-36 "...And when the men of that place recognized Him, they sent out into all that surrounding*

A Vision of Healing

region, brought to Him all who were sick, and begged
Him that they might only touch the hem of His garment.
And as many as touched it were made perfectly well.")

Let me encourage you again in the reading and study of the written Scriptures as you seek to establish your heart and mind concerning healing! The Lord is so willing to show Himself and His truth to everyone who looks for answers in His word!

Whenever you read, ask for revelation to come into your spirit man, to replace in your mind previous mindsets and opinions—anything contrary to the word of the Lord. Again, His word is clear you are transformed (which is what you want to be) by the renewing of your mind! It is a work of the Holy Spirit in you which accomplishes this, and the power or life of the Spirit is in the word of the Scripture. It has the power within it to come to pass if you allow it. Approach the Scripture as life bearing, and with faith that God will do whatever He has committed to do. This is not because He must obey our desires, but because He has obligated Himself to honor His word!

Let the word take root in you as a seed, then pray over (water) it, and guard it from being stolen or negated by contrary circumstance and situations (Matthew 13:3-23). Set the guard from the beginning, because this passage suggests the enemy WILL come to steal the word of truth, that new revelation you have received. Don't be caught off guard. Understand there is persecution for the sake of the word, and because of it (Mark 4:17). You will have to stand firm concerning what you now believe.

Chapter Seven: Grasping Hold

I am very grateful for the Word of Faith movement and those ministries and individuals who taught the Body of Christ how to receive from God by believing His word and trusting in Him! The Lord was restoring something through them, and they obeyed Him to bring forth their portion. The faith movement reminded us of the biblical foundation and our rightful heritage concerning faith. We have learned to look into God's word, locate His promises, and put our trust in them. We have learned to activate our measure of faith, the faith deposit already within us, and put it to use to receive what we or others need. We use faith to cause heavenly things to be released to earth. We also learned to speak the word aloud so that the word of God can be created! Much of the material I studied in the early scramble to understand healing came from teachers in this movement of faith! I honor the role they have had, and appreciate the revelation they have gifted to us all!

One such revelation that markedly aided my search for healing was understanding the difference between belief and faith. The difference is critical for receiving any promise from the Lord.

A Vision of Healing

Faith is essential for receiving because faith is the substance of what you hope for (Hebrews 11:1)! This word says if you have faith you actually already have the thing for which you are hoping—only in the spirit realm first, and then in the natural. The Bible says your faith IS the thing—then the thing appears where you can see it, touch it, and hold it in your hand!

But faith is vastly different than merely believing something is true! When we are in a condition of faith there is a trust element not present in mere belief. We know this from discussions of salvation, where we are clear in our understanding that demons believe in Jesus (and shudder because of His presence; James 2:19), but certainly do not put their trust in Him for salvation.

Faith has an action element that cannot be ignored, because faith without works is dead (James 2:20, 26). Genuine faith will act. You won't have to work up this activity, or pretend. When you have faith, you will just do things that have faith in them. When I disposed of my medications, it wasn't to prove something to God. (That's a good way to lose your life!) The week after the church gathering where I heard the "Today" message, I decided I was meant to believe I was well. I've never taken medication for that disease since. My testimony is that I knew I could take that step because I knew He would catch me. I knew that I could do it, so I did! I have always believed I received about 90% of my manifested healing at that time.

Faith reaches for the promise and grasps hold. Here is how we do it:

> So Jesus answered and said to them, "Have faith
> in God. ²³For assuredly, I say to you, whoever says
> to this mountain, 'Be removed and be cast into the

Wendy Fair Waterson

sea,' and does not doubt in his heart, but believes that those things he says will be done, he will have whatever he says.²⁴Therefore I say to you, whatever things you ask when you pray, believe that you receive them, and you will have them. Mark 11:22-24

Very early in my Holy Spirit instructional on healing He taught me about this word "receive" (verse 24).

It is important to know how to do it, because when you pray a prayer that asks the Lord for anything, you are going to need to believe that you receive it in order to have it come to you!

This word "receive" means to grasp hold of forcefully, just like you would if you were taking something away from someone—which is interesting because God is actually freely giving healing away! I believe He is simply saying, "Grab hold, and don't let go!" He knows the enemy will try to steal it. He knows there will be warfare. He wants you to take the thing from Him, and not lose your grip!

The word "receive"[5] in Mark 11:24 is actually, intriguingly, the same Greek word as the phrase translated "take away" in Matthew 5:40-41, *"If anyone wants to sue you and **take away** your tunic, let him have your cloak also. And whoever compels you to go one mile, go with him two."*[6]

---

5. Strong's Exhaustive Concordance, #2983, "receive."

6. Tracing the word to the Matthew passage must be done with a concordance which lists occurrences of the word take individually with their corresponding numbers and definitions. Newer versions group all occurrences together, and the distinctiveness of each usage is lost. It is a great study to discover the other things the Word of God indicates are to be taken hold of in this passionate way.

A Vision of Healing

What kind of picture does this passage paint for you? I see the person who wants to sue another over their tunic and take it away as a highly intense individual! He or she very much wants the tunic, and insists on having it! They're willing to take you to court for it. There is a determination about their attitude. The Lord says, "It's ok to be intensely determined about receiving My good gifts!" He WANTS us to appropriate them. He encourages us to aggressively pursue them. He isn't holding back anything from us that has been promised in His word. Sometimes I think He's asking, "OK, does anybody actually want anything?"

I have a Holy Spirit word to encourage His people to also "go to court" for what we desire from heaven! Not in the sense of suing people for things, but certainly to petition the throne of God and the courts of heaven for all that is rightfully ours through Jesus Christ! Make no mistake, there is a reality in which the Lord delights to have Jesus' joint heirs, His heavenly family, appear boldly before the throne to obtain His blessings (Hebrews 4:16)!

I will testify that throughout my healing journey there were many days where I experienced various degrees of suffering and learned to insist on my healing! I would say those exact words out loud. "I'm going to have to insist that I'm healed today." I knew I was not twisting God's arm, but rather demanding my healing from the opposing side who always tried to dissuade me in it. More times than I can count, when I insisted, the pain would fall away and I could do that day the things I needed to do as a wife, a mom, and a minister.

I sense the Lord is right now looking for people who will believe and receive. He is searching for someone who will take

Him at His word! As Scripture says, He is watching over the earth, seeking people to whom He can show Himself strong (2 Chronicles 16:9)! These are the ones described as "loyal to Him." I believe these are the ones who believe what He says and actually honor what He has said. They put their faith in Him!

Pursue your promise! When you pray for something you know is God's will, believe He is giving it to you, and it will materialize. Sooner or later you will see and touch it!

Speak the Word in Faith!

As you see the truth revealed through scripture, begin to declare what the Lord has shown to you! Just as God created (and still creates) by the word that He speaks, so also He is able to create through any word of His that you speak!

I say "able to create" because it is necessary to speak the word in faith, and a created work won't happen without it. Someone's got to speak in faith on earth in order to have something from heaven created on this plane!

If declaring seems awkward at first, just begin to release. Practice. You will find it easy to speak out the word in which you really believe; but if you don't believe at first, faith comes by hearing! Say it until you DO believe it! This is an effective strategy based on spiritual principles.

Sooner or later you will actually speak the Scripture or revelation as a statement of fact. You are now speaking it into the atmosphere in order for the Spirit to move upon it. His power will cause the word to create, and be created. Just as Holy Spirit hovered over the void before creation of the world awaiting the

A Vision of Healing

Word of God, so now He awaits the word coming forth through you, ready to cause it to come to pass!

If you speak the word about healing mixed with faith, the fruit of it can be created, and healing will come to you! The Lord will surely perform it!

Chapter Eight: The Wholeness Principle

Having our minds renewed concerning healing is a process. It may be short, or it may take awhile! But if you enter with an open, submitted heart and follow the revelation to its end you come to a revelation of wholeness!

As I read the Scriptures, prayed, listened, and heard, somewhere along the way I realized the Lord and I were no longer talking just about healing, or healings, but a lasting "divine health," or living in a place of His fullness of life manifest in our body that would move me beyond sickness and disease and into a manifestation of His life throughout my entire being; body, soul and spirit.

Returning to 1 Peter 2:24 *"By whose stripes you were healed,"* it is easy to see why wholeness belongs to us in Jesus! Having effected our restoration to the Father, Jesus has bought back for us what had been lost—perfection.

We are not only "fixed" when we are healed, we are actually *completely restored* to perfection! It's not as though we need to expect to retain some stiffness in our knee, or shortness of breath, or ability to do things we did before. I would contend even the scars of injuries can be removed with the fullness of restoration that God has accomplished in Jesus, and I have heard these kinds of testimonies. Some may disagree on this point, but I believe the Spirit is calling us to abandon what we have known and receive greater degrees of revelation. I'll receive again with you! If we are fully restored we can expect complete wholeness to be renewed in and around us, for that is how we were with Father God in the beginning!

There are many Scriptures that speak of wholeness and being made whole. Jesus declared wholeness over individuals in some of His healings. To the blind man He said, *"Go thy way, thy faith hath made thee whole"* (Mark 10:52, KJV). Matthew 15:31 describes many people being healed of various maladies--and made whole, to the amazement of the crowds who were witnesses! As I sought the Lord concerning healing over years, I began to believe God's provision was actually for our spirit, soul and body—our entire man. Father God addressed the brokenness of our sin and our sickness in the same way—through His provision in Jesus Christ! The provision in Jesus is full. Nothing is left out!

If our restoration is full, we will have nothing needful lacking at all. Receiving this revelation by faith will release a manifestation of divine health in every aspect of our lives!

Now Death Is Defeated

There is more to our salvation in Jesus than most people say—that we have forgiveness of sin and a place in heaven someday. There is more to salvation than many who perceive that it includes physical healing may even have understood. From the early days of my healing study with the Lord I knew this must ultimately be true. The glorious thread of healing leads to one more place. What started as an inkling, a holy suspicion, eventually became a compelling conviction. The revelation of what has been provided in Jesus Christ culminates in the realization that there is no more death!

*My mouth shall tell **of** Your righteousness And Your **salvation** all **the day**, For I do not know **their** limits. Psalm 71:15*

The righteousness and the salvation of God that He has extended to us are more awesome than we have the ability to describe in words, and they absolutely exceed our ability to comprehend them with our human minds! David acknowledged he did not know the extent to which these blessings reached, the fullness of their work, or their "limits." Several other translations of this verse speak of these gifts of righteousness and salvation, saying we do not know their "numbers." All that is included in these gifts is more than we could count, or wrap our minds around to understand. In our hearts we have many times truly not known what we have received!

This is why we need help from Holy Spirit! He reveals what we could otherwise never know, and gives us language to talk about it. Receiving heavenly revelation requires a humble, seeking heart, willing to have assumptions changed through divine insight. We do well when we come to the Lord with a willingness to lay down our opinions. It also helps to be willing to be mocked for your radical God-ideas. Remember, just as in high school algebra, "radical" means "pertaining to the root"—and in this case the root means Jesus. Be as radical as you like!

It is the revelation of complete restoration to our Creator God that brings understanding about deliverance from death. Quite simply, if we are fully restored to our original state with Him, death must by definition have been removed from us. For those who have been restored to God through Jesus, there can be no more death.

A full study called "No More Death," lays out the case for this conclusion, and has been released in our local church body twice. I anticipate putting it in print, and hope it can inspire the Body of Christ, along with similar revelation through others hearing the same thing, to move up higher in the spirit, operating in greater authority through revelation of our position in Him! Without doubt, we will be moving into Christ in such a way in the coming days that we will no longer live with an expectation of death. Praise our God!!!

Divine Health Through Divine Wisdom

Once we are open to receiving wholeness from the Lord He begins to release wisdom from heaven to bring us into a new reality of divine health. You may experience this if you pray for healing. He will begin to make adjustments to you to help you be healed--and stay that way for life!

I was personally given information from Him at various times about ways of conducting myself aligned with His wisdom. They were practical steps I sensed through the Spirit He wanted me to take. Heeding and following these kinds of instructions is important! His ways are perfect! I saw enormous benefit from taking them seriously and following through. Many times, if full transformation eluded me, Father God would send help through some practical step that would bring me marked relief. One way He did this was through words of knowledge (1 Corinthians 12) pointing out the roots from which some of my physical problems stemmed. With this information, helpful solutions could be discerned. I have learned to pay attention to the voice of the Spirit! I both ask questions and expect answers I need for life!

In this manner, while receiving that last 5% healing manifestation, I was shown I had celiac disease, or gluten allergy. I had not known this condition "ran" in my family line. I felt the Lord directed me to stop eating wheat specifically for a year, and I felt much better, with much less pain in my joints than before. The characteristic rash associated with it left me. Then as I believed God for healing of this specific condition I began to add wheat back to my diet little by little. I have no symptoms of celiac disease to this date, and wheat and gluten do not produce the inflammation they seemed to before.

I want to encourage YOU with this, because there may be times you need specific wisdom while you are having your mind transformed concerning healing. It feels disappointing at first, but God knows best. His concern is getting you well in any way He can. His priority is delivering you out of pain and suffering.

Peas, Menopause and Canola Oil

The Lord delights me with His ways! Words of knowledge and of wisdom frequently come as simple words and phrases, softly spoken to the consciousness. Sometimes they come as an image, like a flash vision. They cause us to say, "I get the picture!"

Over time I have heard from Father God through the Spirit on many different subjects in this manner, including things like national security issues! In the last two week I have heard each one of the 7 current presidential candidates' names in the

A Vision of Healing

2016 presidential primaries race, so I have prayed for them all! I consider all such communications to be first for purposes of intercession, and second to be acted upon if so directed.

It's always important to pray over what you perceive to be a directional word from God. Prayer can be made to seek confirmation of the word you have heard. Pray and ask what the Lord means by what He has shared with you. He tells us things for a reason. Always ask why! Many missteps are made through wrong interpretations, so waiting for confirmation is important. It is a good idea to get counsel from trusted, godly individuals who hear the Lord if you sense you need to have someone else view the information with a fresh spiritual eye.

Whether heavenly wisdom comes as an impression, or as a word you would swear was spoken aloud right next to you, all can be regarded as precious and able to change our circumstances if heeded! When my body was especially fatigued a few years ago, I had a vision in a dream of a large bowl of peas. That's all, just peas! My understanding was I must have been low on iron. An easy change to my diet was a quick fix!

Another word of knowledge came very clearly to me at the beginning of 2013 when the Spirit broke into my consciousness as I was getting dressed one day with the word "menopause."

"Is that for ME?" I thought.

It was. I won't bother to give many details, but this was a needed word for me! It became a caution when my body shifted sharply where my metabolism was concerned, and I had to purpose to watch what I ate in a way I had ever had to before. I understand now what it is like for people who say they can just look at desserts and gain weight! After quickly gaining 20 pounds

Wendy Fair Waterson

I applied myself to eating with more wisdom from the Lord, after a new pattern, and was able to see my weight begin to shift back to a healthier level.

In 2014 another remarkable prophetic word came to me during a time a strange rash appeared across my chest. I had never seen anything like it. It was extremely itchy, and one of those things that cause you to say, "This is making me crazy!"

After nearly 3 months enduring in this situation, I finally realized I hadn't asked the Lord for help! I immediately prayed for the rash to be removed. Literally within minutes I heard the Spirit say, *"canola oil."*

It was time to pray for an interpretation via the Spirit, because I didn't know whether the phrase "canola oil" was indication to eat it, or to avoid it! In this case, after praying I believed the Lord was impressing me that I should no longer use canola oil. Upon reflection I realized I had not really been exposed to it for very long, but had recently switched to a canola blend for cooking. After further prayer I heard a second word to confirm my decision to remove the oil from our household, and it had to do with timing. I distinctly heard *"in six weeks."*

Was this right? I timed my separation from canola oil, including in all purchase packaged items. Exactly six weeks later all that remained was one tiny head-of-a-pin sized spot where the rash had been—and the next day it was completely gone! I am certain this was His instruction in answer to my seeking a solution, as I accidently ate some canola later, and immediately got a few spots back!

What an awesome God! That's how good He is, and how concerned Father God is for our welfare! I will testify I know for sure that He cares about each detail of our lives, from the smallest to the biggest. Certainly if He will talk to us about peas, He will engage us concerning a much needed healing or other urgent matter!

During the time I was intensely ill I had a "revelation" about parking spaces that illustrates this point, though admittedly in in a rather simplistic way. I'll call it the "Parking Space Theory."

Can we all admit we have prayed to the Lord for a parking space when we needed one? We even asked for a "good" parking space. And we have testimonies (we've probably either given or heard in church) of how God responded to provide just what we needed! I am not implying there is a single thing wrong with praying this prayer, by the way. However, my humble theory is that if the Lord answered a casual parking space request with a "yes" even *once* for any person throughout all time, then obviously He says "yes" to an urgent request for healing!

> Look at **the birds of the air**, *for* **they** *neither sow nor reap nor gather into barns; yet your heavenly Father feeds* **them**. *Are you not* **of** *more value than* **they**? *Matthew 6:26*

My hope is that we will be finished with thinking our heavenly Father is distant and disengaged. Let's also never imagine He doesn't care to heal us and guide us into a life of full restoration and peace! He is highly invested in us, having given Jesus. Then He lavished on us every gift through Him!

Getting You to the Place You Can Be Healed

The Father supplies ALL our need, large or small, demonstrating His desire for us to be whole in every aspect of our lives. He patiently works with us to unravel our tangled life situations, including our health problems, until they are completely resolved.

If necessary, the Spirit will work on your soul first, in order to get you healed. Issues of sin or forgiveness may be dealt with. I do not find these to be definitive prerequisites for physical healing, though certainly they are of a high priority. People who are totally unsaved have been healed, and the Lord does not indicate He requires them to be sanctified first. Still, always be open to His intervention in the realm of your mind, will and emotions. He knows if an issue will block YOU from receiving your healing. He will know when these issues will need to be dealt with at the outset. He is trying to get your healing to you!

I have seen the Lord work intensely with people over months and years in order to accomplish this. He is giving each one their best chance at receiving. Some need their soul to prosper to a certain degree before they can even begin to be healed. The word says that as our soul prospers, we also prosper in our bodies (3 John 1:2). This Scripture says He desires that to be the case! For our soul to prosper, each part of it must come into peace. These kinds of inner healing are necessary for wholeness, and can significantly aid many physical restoration processes.

At all times remember God is on your side. He gave His only Son for your freedom from every kind of disability. He holds NOTHING back from you!

Chapter Nine: A Vision of Healing is a Revelation of Jesus!

M y healing has been a journey with God.

As I write to you I am feeling very well! I have no pain except occasionally in my hands. Today I got up with zero stiffness, did a cardio routine with weights for 40 minutes, worked around the house, and later walked briskly for 65 minutes—nearly 3 miles. I take no medications, though I do use some herbal supplements I felt the Lord showed to me.

Nevertheless, the fact remains, overall I have been a bit of a slow healer. That last 5% manifestation has only come over time and through bring very honest before the Lord about my difficulty! I have said to Him I am sorry I have at times not fully taken Him at His word. I have doubted His word to me. I know when I am in doubt, because at those times I am not resting in my heart and mind. At times I've been like a child learning float in water. Even with someone nearby to hold me, I have struggled to relax and lean back. Time and time again I have jerked back up and begun to sink!

Faith is knowing you are safe! It is assurance and peace! It really is knowing you have the thing for which you've asked before you ever see it! Admitting we have doubt is a first step in having our faith grow.

As time has gone by the Lord has worked with me in my places of unbelief, giving me other options for relief, and always encouraging me by His word. I have chosen to walk this way of healing. It really has been like walking on the water! I didn't have to choose to do it, but I wanted to. And when I said, "If it is You, Lord, bid me to come," like Peter did, He held out His hand to me. Whenever I started sinking, He lifted me up!

Twenty years since the diagnosis in 1995, my heavenly Father has honored my prayer to change me until I can fully receive! I have learned much from Him. I have considered myself to be at the Lord's feet, taught of Him like Mary. In that time both my understanding and my faith have grown. In fact, over the years I have instructed many concerning healing, particularly in my role as a pastor and teacher. I have prayed for many, declaring healing over them as released by the Lord to do so. I have seen sickness recovered from many times, diseases and injuries healed, and much preventative provision released which has kept many from becoming ill. My family has enjoyed a degree of health that I would call remarkable.

In the midst of all this I have known myself to be in an ongoing process of receiving revelation of what I have been given in Jesus Christ. Even in light of all I have shared in the earlier chapters of this book, I have desired my own understanding to be made deeper, and ever more complete. I have wanted to walk in a fullness of revelation and of provision, and then of release to others of God's healing and delivering power! I have distinctly known He has wanted to truly give me His own mind concerning all He is to us and has done in bringing us into Christ.

The Lord hears our genuine prayers for answers! He is willing to teach us what we need to know. I prayed and asked for help once again.

> *Call to Me, and I will answer you, and show you great and mighty things, which you do not know. Jeremiah 33:3*

It was November 22, 2008 that there came a new release to me from heaven. By this time I had seen and heard many supernatural things through the Spirit of God, some of which have been described in this book. This was like nothing I had experienced before. It was a vision of healing!

Waking from the Dream Encounter

I left the light of heavenly glory that had filled my vision in sleep, but in my bedroom the Spirit was still distinctly present. It was captivating to be close to the Lord God and to have Him speak this way through Holy Spirit. His voice was so lovely, and His presence so precious!

An energy that I could feel physically and tangibly was with me in the room, like a vibration in the air all around me. I was not moving. I remained very still; but I felt so alive! I was full of excitement and amazement at what, and who, I had encountered! I lay there thanking Him out loud for what had taken place, full of joy. I praised the Lord!

A Vision of Healing

This vision must have been in answer to my request! I remembered how in recent weeks I had been asking God again for help concerning healing. I had been praying to see a fullness of restoration in my body—and I had been newly petitioning the Lord concerning my aging eyes. It was thrilling to have new revelation of any kind concerning healing to look at and pray through!

But a sense of puzzlement was in my heart. I was very happy; but oddly uneasy. I didn't like it.

Playing the scene from the beach over again in my mind, I felt incredulous--truly mystified. Had the Spirit of the Lord just said to me what I thought I had heard? Had He really said, *"I'm going to fix that"?* Yes, without a doubt He had looked into my imperfect eyes and made that statement, one hand on either side of my face. It was unforgettable. He had said that, and nothing else. Then I awoke.

In my bed I tested my eyes expectantly, holding my hand close to my face, trying out my capacity to see up close. I knew I had received *something* from God—but my vision close up was the same. It was very blurry. I looked across the room, trying out my distance vision which had been only slightly impaired. I was certain there was a difference.

I would come to know I did experience a healing, as I could now see perfectly at a distance. On my next visit to the eye doctor I was told my bifocals were essentially not needed. "Really I've made the distance portion with no prescription," he said. But reading was still a problem. In that regard I could see no better— and I couldn't believe it! I was astounded Holy Spirit Himself laid hands on me, addressed that very issue, yet I was not made immediately perfect!

My dilemma was clearly more internal than anything, since in many ways reading glasses are not a big deal; however, it still drove me immediately to seek the Lord in prayer! To me it was vitally important to know why the Spirit said, *"I'm going to fix that!"* when by now I knew beyond a doubt that healing is for today--it's for NOW, and has effectively already been given to us! Why would the Spirit of God, the God of Today healing, refer to a healing as something He would do in the future? I knew there had to be a distinct reason. Everything God does is deliberate and for specific purpose. What was the meaning of this act on His part?

During the next week I rehearsed over and over again what had happened in the dream. By now I officially referred to it as an encounter! I believed that it truly happened in the spirit realm; that is, Holy Spirit actually met me in a spiritual place in order to speak directly to me concerning healing! Another thing I now believed was that this experience from the Lord was really about much more than my eyes. It was just dawning in my mind--but deep within my spirit I knew--this encounter was going to birth a new revelation of healing that would take me further into wholeness than I had previously come. I knew I was about to be freer than ever before.

Over the next weeks and months the Lord taught me concerning my vision of healing. What He spoke came in three parts and at three different times. Each time I received more healing!

Vision Revelation Part One: Holy Spirit Reveals Jesus!

The Lord is very specific in His actions, and very purposed in all He does. We can be sure that every word of His is significant, and each detail of any dream or vision or encounter is key. Nothing in God is wasted.

A Vision of Healing

As I prayed and asked about His intentions in the encounter I felt He wanted me to consider a question very answerable by Scripture, *"What does the Holy Spirit do?"* The Lord was having me focus on the work and ministry of His Holy Spirit, and how He, the Spirit, would do what He said in my dream--"fix that."

Here are three foundational things we know about Holy Spirit through the written word of God (there are many more): 1) We are born again by the Spirit, 2) We are sealed by the Spirit, 3) Holy Spirit reveals the things of God.

Holy Spirit reveals the things of God because there are things we could never know about Him without Him showing them to us! They are deep in Him. Holy Spirit opens them to us and helps us understand these mysteries! Some of these hidden things in God are the things we have been given by Him! How sad if we were never to know! But Holy Spirit graciously shows and tells us.

But as it is written:
"Eye has not seen, nor ear heard,
Nor have entered into the heart of man
The things which God has prepared for those who
love Him."[c]
[10]But God has revealed them to us through His Spirit. For the Spirit searches all things, yes, the deep things of God. [11]For what man knows the things of a man except the spirit of the man which is in him? Even so no one knows the things of God except the Spirit of God. [12]Now we have received, not the spirit of the world, but the Spirit who is from God, that we might know the things that have been freely given to us by God. I Corinthians 2:10-12

Wendy Fair Waterson

I am convinced out of all the things of God He is meant to reveal, Holy Spirit's favorite is Jesus! Holy Spirit draws us to the knowledge of salvation in Jesus. He shows us our need for Him. He testifies of what He has done. He is the faithful witness to the truth of who Jesus is!

> *This is He who came by water and blood—Jesus Christ; not only by water, but by water and blood. And it is **the Spirit** who bears witness, because **the Spirit** is truth. I John 5:6*

It is by the Spirit we can know He is Lord.

> *...no one can say that Jesus is Lord **except by the Holy Spirit**. I Corinthians 12:3*

Again, in Ephesians 3:3-5 Paul says that by revelation from the Spirit he was shown the mystery of Christ.

Finally, the greatest privilege we have been given by God is the ability to be transformed into the image of Christ—by the power of the Spirit!!!

> *But we all, with unveiled face, beholding as in a mirror the glory of the Lord, are being transformed into the same image from glory to glory, just as by the Spirit of the Lord. 2 Corinthians 3:18*

The Lord reminded me of all these things out of my encounter on the beach. It was a vision of the Holy Spirit, and a vision about healing, because He declared He would provide healing of my vision. But I have come to know that, in truth, when He said, *"I'm going to fix that,"* He meant He would cause me to truly

71

see clearly spiritually first. The vision was a statement from God that revelation was coming that would help me to really see and know the truth. **The vision became a promise that He would show me Jesus!**

When I considered how it is Holy Spirit's assignment to reveal the things of God and to show us Jesus Christ, I understood my dream and the statement He had made. A vision of healing is a revelation of Jesus Christ! Holy Spirit knew that when I saw Jesus clearly I would receive healing fully--healing of my vision, but also of everything else. He knew that as my spiritual vision was healed, and as I saw Jesus accurately and fully by revelation, I would be like Him--whole and complete--for I would see Him as He is!!!! And this is what He promised to do! Praise and glory to God!!!

> *Beloved, now we are children of God; and it has not yet been revealed what we shall be, but we know that when **He is** revealed, we shall be like **Him**, for we shall **see Him as He is**. 1 John 3:2*

Vision Revelation Part Two: How Great He Is; How Powerful!

I have been in seasons of praying over the vision. I welcome the Lord to speak again and again into what I saw and experienced, as He shares with me from His heart the things I need to know. Holy Spirit is teaching me. He is helping me to see Jesus!

Very recently He did this by asking me two specific questions. The answers reveal more about the Lord Jesus and confirm again the fullness of His provision of salvation. They are revelations that have now moved me into greater manifestation of healing in my body and total divine health for my life.

Wendy Fair Waterson

Holy Spirit Asked, "How Complete was His Work?"

This question was released deep in my spirit. I sensed Holy Spirit speak again as a distinct impression in my mind, interrupting my chain of thought about more mundane things as He had now often done before.

"How complete was His work?"

As always, I was delighted to hear from Holy Spirit! My heart was stirred to attention, and I listened expectantly, with excitement for what was to come. I sensed this conversation was in answer to my prayers for understanding, and that this was an important question He expected me to answer. Clearly it was a reference to Jesus. I surmised was about to go "back to school" to learn more about My Savior and Healer and the vision on the beach! Holy Spirit was about to show Him to me again!

To answer the question I began to reflect and meditate upon the work of Jesus on the cross. What, exactly, was the extent of the work? What, precisely, was the nature of His accomplishment? My mind searched the Scriptures accounts, settling on Isaiah 53, from which Holy Spirit had previously instructed me.

According to Isaiah 53:4-5, Jesus' sacrifice leaves no need unaddressed.

> *Surely He has borne our griefs and carried our sorrows; yet we esteemed Him stricken, smitten by God, and afflicted. But He was wounded for our transgressions, He was bruised for our iniquities; the chastisement for our peace was upon Him, and by His stripes we are healed.*

A Vision of Healing

From this account we know the sacrifice addressed and took all of our griefs, sorrows, transgressions, iniquities, lack of peace and brokenness. He has borne them, carried them, been wounded for them, bruised for them, chastised for them and beaten because of them. Again, the result was the release of our complete healing! Nothing has been left out. The effect of the work is paramount and thoroughly exhaustive. There is no malady or dysfunction that is not covered by this list, brought under the power of the healing we discovered earlier was defined as wholeness in every way!

As I rehearsed these truths again and meditated upon them, the Spirit urged me to see more! Next I saw again the provision through Jesus' resurrection. I saw it afresh, although I had viewed it many times before.

Paul prayed we would have the Spirit of wisdom and revelation so that we could know, *"what is the exceeding greatness of His power toward us who believe, according to the working of His mighty power* [20] *which He worked in Christ when He raised Him from the dead."* (Ephesians 1:19-20a)

Jesus was raised up with the keys of hades and of death, victorious over every work of the enemy. His resurrection and his entrance again into heavenly places raised us up to that identical place of victory, provision and authority! It was the seal on the work of the cross, for Jesus' resurrection effectively made His one-time sacrifice good for all--forever! His blood speaks salvation for all mankind for all time because He rose and took His own blood before the Father, placing it on the mercy seat where it declares His work for all eternity!

A revelation of how complete the work of Jesus on the cross was, and the fullness of the provision through His sacrifice, brings great reassurance concerning healing! All things are covered, and the work is finished!

Holy Spirit Asked, "Have You Considered His Greatness?"

Two days after the first question about the vision came to me I clearly heard the Spirit ask a second question. This time it was more than an impression, but spoken once again in that manner words of knowledge can come—as though someone is talking near me, while the voice is clearly heard in my mind.

"Have you considered His greatness?"

Again, I knew this meant I needed to! I went back to Ephesians 1:19. This time I believed Holy Spirit wanted to highlight the *"exceeding greatness of His power."*

To consider this power is to become acquainted with strength and ability greater than that possessed by any other being or created thing. It is the power of God, who is all-powerful! Holy Spirit knows that a revelation of this great power excelling far above all others will cause us to know the healing that is in Christ overwhelms the power of any sickness that could exist in our bodies! The power of God will overcome whatever opposes Him. His strength rules over all!

This emphasis of the Spirit caused me to recall the first few years in healing circles amongst people who professed that God was willing to heal, but who then seemed to always be wonder when it was going to happen. And one of them used to be me! However, a conviction about the greatness of His power removes us from imagining a sickness could ever endure in spite of His ability! Acknowledging that His power is greater causes us to see that the devil cannot withstand Him.

Suddenly we realize the healing He is willing to do can even be instantaneous, if we would believe! Perhaps we can move into a reality of speaking healing and believing to see it immediately manifest—if we believe in the greatness of His power!

This great power of God lavished on Jesus raised Him from the dead, and is now invested in Him, in His presence, His name and His blood. It is for us! We access it through seeing Him and taking hold of its reality. By trusting Him we receive His great power expressed into our otherwise hopeless situations. His power is more than enough to break forth for our healing! The power of the resurrection is the power that now heals and delivers. It is the power that works IN US, working IN US the provisions of the cross!

"Thank you, Holy Spirit," I said.

Vision Revelation Part Three: "This is My Beloved Son"

Revisiting the vision in my thoughts, again in my bed, I recalled how Holy Spirit came down to me as a dove. Partly asleep, and partly awake, another question floated through my consciousness.

"Why did I choose to appear to you first in the vision as a dove?"

I had assumed the Spirit came as a dove so I would know beyond a doubt who He was. The idea of Holy Spirit had always first brought this image to my mind. I felt He appeared as a dove so I would know Him as the Spirit before He transformed into the unfamiliar spirit with a human-like face. There may have been an element of that, but there was more. There was a deeper meaning behind this decision of the Lord to manifest His Spirit as the dove.

As I meditated on the Lord's newest question, He reminded me of the account of Jesus' baptism and what had transpired when the Spirit descended upon Jesus like a dove. As the Spirit rested upon Him, the Father spoke and said, *"This is my beloved son, in whom I am well pleased!"* (Matthew 3:17)

This is what the Spirit showed me next: Whoever else He touches, Holy Spirit always comes and rests upon the Father's sons and daughters!

The knowledge of Christ through Scripture that says that we are joint heirs with Jesus of everything the Father has given to Him filled me in a new way! There was indication of vast heavenly provision, and Holy Spirit confirming that sons and daughters of God are not lacking, but are possessors of all things that are given to Jesus as His inheritance! They receive *"all things that have to do with life and godliness!"* (2 Peter 1:3) Surely, He said, Jesus was firstborn among many brethren, and we had been granted a share with Him—a right to all that the Father has!

I sensed strongly the Father emphasizing His great love for me. He was saying it was equal to the love He had for His Son Jesus! I felt Him bringing deep revelation of how completely I was accepted into His embrace as His very own child.

This is what I sensed the Father say: "You are My beloved, and I am pleased with you! It is the privilege of My sons and daughters to receive My Spirit just as Jesus did. You are received by Me just as He was; you are as blessed by Me as well. Walk in the reality of My presence and provision in the same way! This is for all My children!"

A Vision of Healing

In that place of His love I knew I was whole. I was convinced if I could carry this love away and live in it, all things would forever be complete in me. What more could I need that wasn't in it? This was the heartbeat of God's presence and His glory spoken of in John 17:22-23 when Jesus said to the Father, *"And the glory which You gave Me I have given them, that they may be one just as We are one: I in them, and You in Me; that they may be made perfect in one, and that the world may know that You have sent Me, and have loved them as You have loved Me."*

I knew Holy Spirit was helping me visualize and to begin to grasp a revelation of oneness with Jesus, and then with the Father, that I had never conceived or understood in this way before.

With every new revelation, Holy Spirit was helping me see more clearly spiritually. As I saw, I was healed!

Chapter Ten: Knowing Him

F rom the beginning of a desperate search for help, through all that has happened since, the greatest contributor to my healing in the end has simply been knowing the Lord! Although He had been part of my life since childhood, in a relationship personal and real, it is clear now that I did not know Him well in very key respects.

I had to seek God to know Him.

> *My son, if you receive my words,*
> *And treasure my commands within you,*
> *²So that you incline your ear to wisdom,*
> *And apply your heart to understanding;*
> *³Yes, if you cry out for discernment,*
> *And lift up your voice for understanding,*
> *⁴If you seek her as silver,*
> *And search for her as for hidden treasures;*
> *⁵Then you will understand the fear of the LORD,*
> *And find the knowledge of God. Proverbs 2:1-5*

Pride will keep us from finding and having revelation of Him. He will not show Himself to those who lift themselves up as though they have no need. The fear of the Lord is the beginning of all wisdom, and this respect and honor for God leads to life (Psalm 111:10; Proverbs 19:23). As the above passage states, it is those who gain an understanding of the fear of the Lord who will find the knowledge of God.

Only when I pressed into God, pursuing Him diligently, did I begin to know the Lord differently. Only by seeking did I find out those things I had never known: His willingness to heal, His ability which is too powerful to fail, the fact that He had no intention of making me wait, and the finality of it all in the work of Jesus! As I encountered Him in various ways our relationship developed a new intimacy. And He was true to His word that if we draw near to Him, He draws near to us! He was unquestionably faithful to the promise. Out of this new relationship of *knowing* I was able to begin to trust Him to be and to do all that He said.

Many testify to receiving healing through the anointing on a gifted minister, some through prayers of faith of the elders of a church, some through the intercession of friends. People have been healed who have not known the Lord a day in their life, and others have been freed from sickness in corporate meetings where the Spirit was powerfully flowing. All of this is wonderful! I believe these authentic stories of healing and deliverance! But knowing God deeply and personally can move you from having to go somewhere to get prayer to walking in wholeness every day of your life! It can change you from a receiver to a releaser of God's truth and His power.

Paul declared he was willing to give up everything else in His life in exchange for knowing God! He said by virtue of his own experience the knowledge of Christ the Lord was an excellent thing.

Wendy Fair Waterson

Yet indeed I also count all things loss for the excellence of the knowledge of Christ Jesus my Lord, for whom I have suffered the loss of all things, and count them as rubbish, that I may gain Christ... Philippians 8:8

In the original Greek the word for "excellence" means that which is *superior, higher, better* and *supreme.* [7]

That is our God! He is higher, and greater, more beautiful, more glorious (Psalm 71:19)—so much so that glory is the definition of His presence (Exodus 33:18-19)! To be with Him is to experience everything that is good and right (Psalm 24:5). To know Him is to know all that is pure, holy love (1 John 4:8). Every good thing comes from Him (James 1:17). Knowing Him brings us into strength, and moves Him to fill us with His power. Eventually we, through knowing Him, become like Him and perform His exploits (Daniel 11:32).

I will testify to you that knowing the Lord is so wonderful He would be enough to satisfy my soul even if I were never physically healed. But praise be to our God! To know God is to know the one who is All in All. To be in Him is to be one with all He is. To know Him is to BE healed! We can't help it! Knowing Him is everything!

---

7. Strong's Exhaustive Concordance, #5242, "excellency."

Conclusion

A fullness has come with each revelation I have received, including from the vision of Holy Spirit on the beach—like a seed that grows and finally produces the harvest it was destined to bear. I received another manifestation, like a sampling of the mature fruit of my healing, during the season I began to write this book.

Reflecting on my journey of healing, I praised God daily for who He is and how He had faithfully answered me and shown me Jesus. I had learned so much that it felt as though I was no longer the same person. So much had shifted. I had blossomed spiritually, become strong in the Lord, and begun to function in His authority in ministry to others. It was evident my health had dramatically improved since the days of crippling pain and lost quality of life. I continued to receive health in my body in every aspect. I felt I was in a process of manifested restoration, and over time all things were being made new!

November 17, 2014 was the eve of my 51st birthday. I was in prayer with some other believers from our apostolic team. As always when we met, we were experiencing the presence of the Lord, expecting to hear from Him.

A Vision of Healing

Although my eyes were closed, I could see us gathered together in the room. It was as though I was lifted above us, granted for a moment a God's-eye view. I saw that Jesus was there. He was present with us in our circle of intercession, just like the Bible says! As we prayed it was as if we were gazing directly at Him through our prayers. He, Himself, was looking back into our eyes with intense passion, great delight, and His always awesome love! In this new vision He looked at me directly, then said authoritatively to us all, *"You are whole!"*

I was surprised, because if He said anything that night I expected it would be something else—perhaps something regarding strategy for our region. That's the kind of meeting it was. But when He said we were whole, I knew that it was right. It was what He should say.

All that Holy Spirit had taught me about Jesus and my healing in Him flooded back upon me that night. Within seconds I somehow viewed a survey of my history, my journey toward healing, and the things He had revealed to me over the last 19 years. I saw that He had spoken to me in so many ways, sent so much help, provided practical solutions, and revolutionized my thinking. I had a renewed mindset.

I thought about the vision which had brought me further into this new reality. I remembered vividly the moment Holy Spirit's eyes burned into mine. Jesus' gaze of fiery love I was seeing now was so like it, and yet different and new.

Holy Spirit had promised to fix my blurred vision when I had seen Him before. He had caused me to see increasingly clearly in the time that had passed, just as He said He would do. But it was by showing me Jesus! The vision of healing had been meant to lead me to begin to truly see HIM. A vision of healing is a vision of Jesus! It is a revelation of Jesus Christ my salvation and deliverance--fully willing and supremely able, embracing me fully into His love and provision, and even into Himself and the glory He has with the Father. This is what Holy Spirit taught me through the vision in the night.

In this new significant moment, I felt I had finally arrived at an important destination.

He said, *"You are whole."* I realized I believed what Jesus had just said. I felt that I knew Him well enough to believe it. I said it back to Him, out loud in the room. Worship music was playing and everyone was praying, and the words I said were not heard by my friends, but I said them anyway into the air.

"We are whole!!!"

Then out of the spirit realm Jesus said to me, *"Now we understand one another! You are whole!"*

....

END

Printed in the United States
By Bookmasters